The illustrations for this book were painted by Gaby Verdooren.
The text type was set in Asbela Eternity. The title font was hand-lettered by Rachel Bostick.

ISBN: 978-1956712162 (Hardcover)
ISBN: 978-1956712179 (E-Book)

Library of Congress publication data available upon request.

First printing edition 2024. Printed in China.
Cover design and typesetting by Misty Black.

Moon Dust Press
Austin, Texas
United States of America
www.moondustpress.com

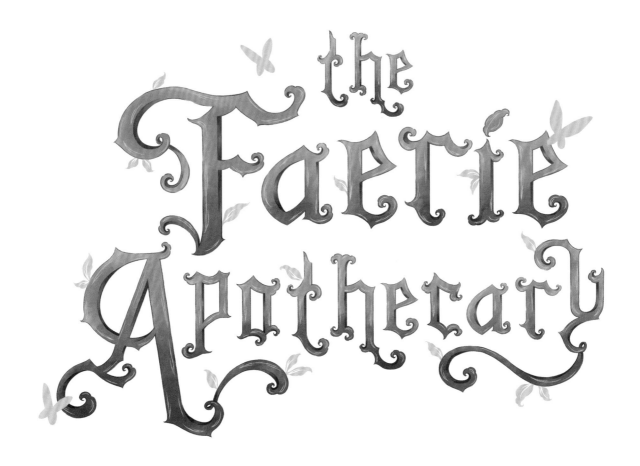

the Faerie Apothecary

Written by
Andrea Stein

Illustrated by
Gaby Verdooren

For the women who inspire
me everyday;
Mom, Nora, Jenn, and Deb
- GV

To the witches of Austin
for all the magic they
spread
- AS

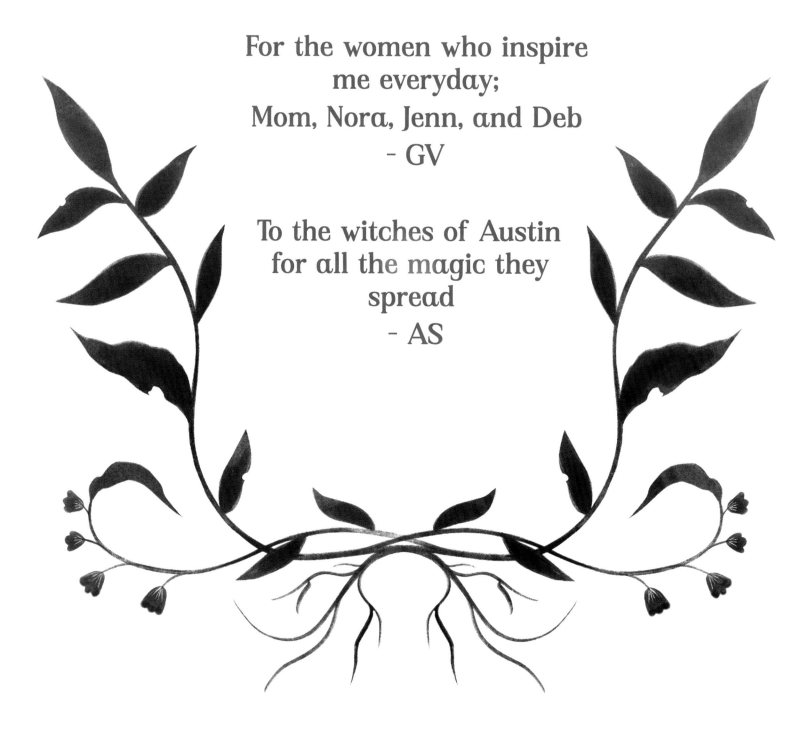

A note from the faeries:

Plants can make magical medicines, but not all plants are safe for humans to touch! Be sure to ask a grown-up before you use any herbal remedies.

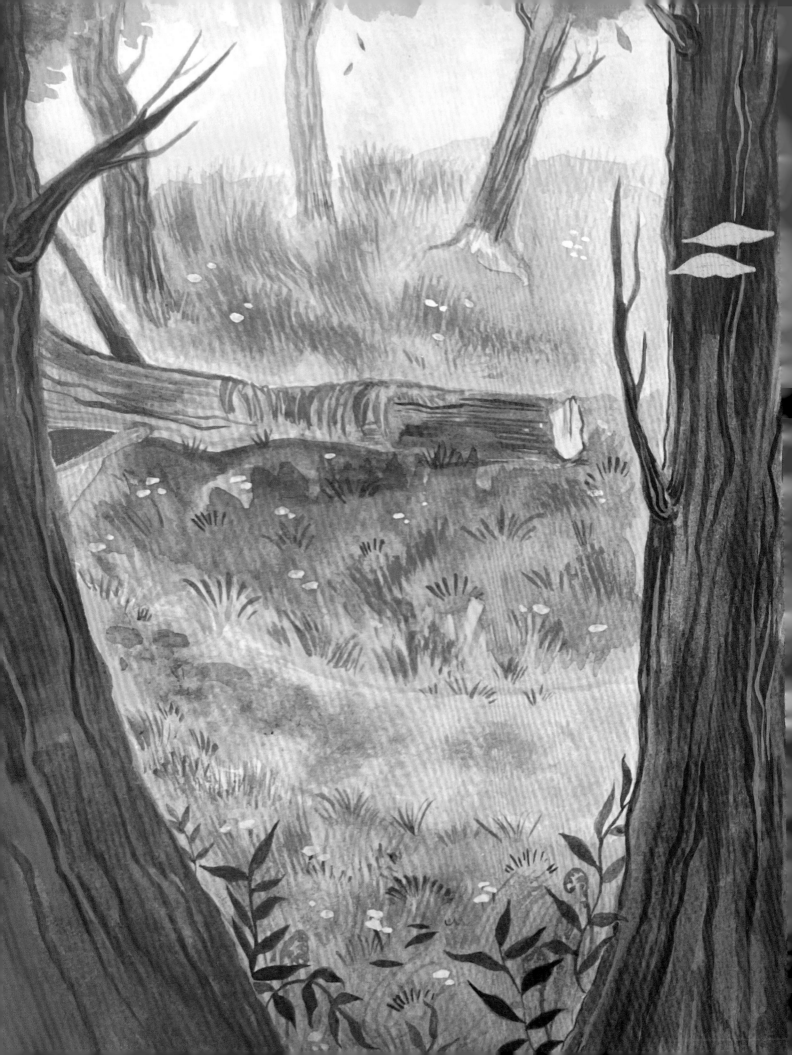

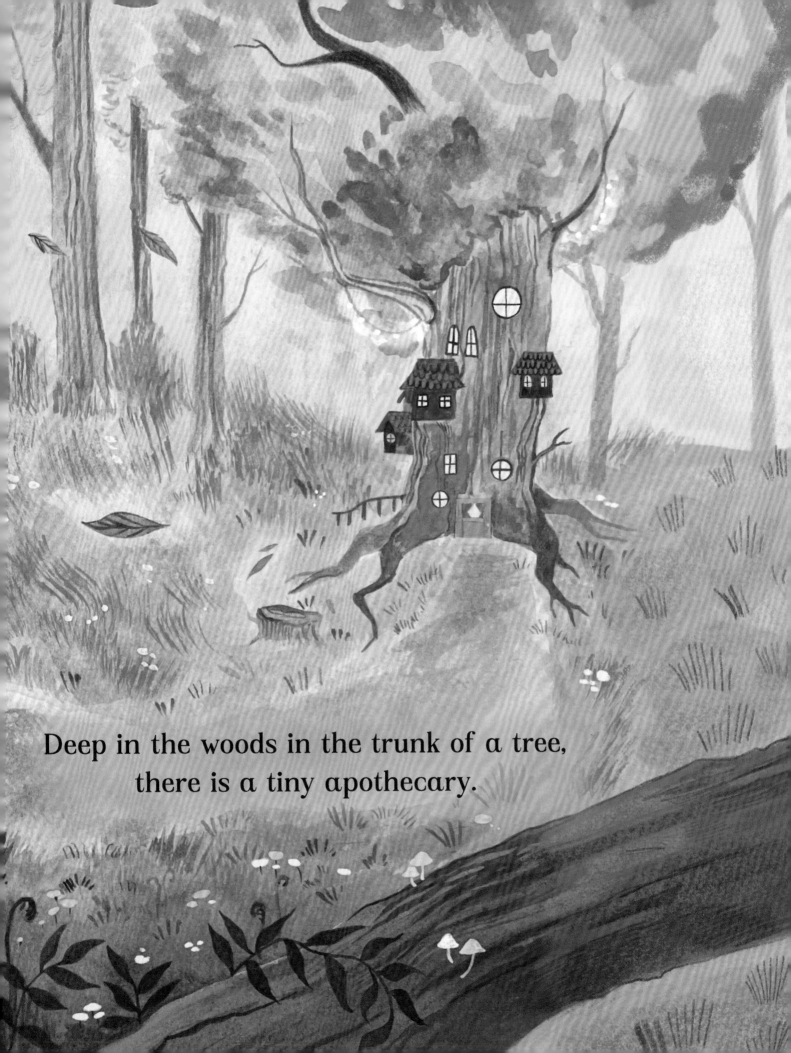

Deep in the woods in the trunk of a tree,
there is a tiny apothecary.

Jingle the bell and then knock on the door

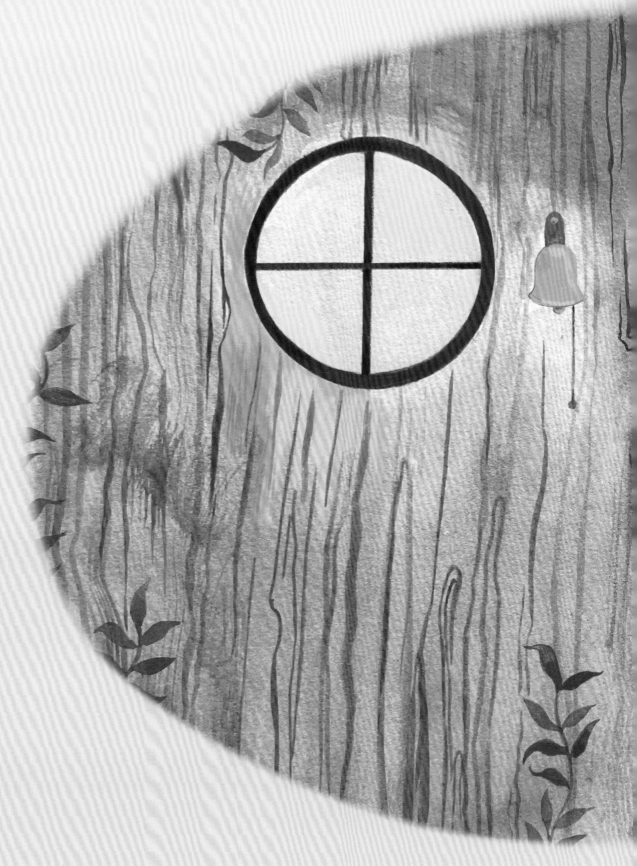

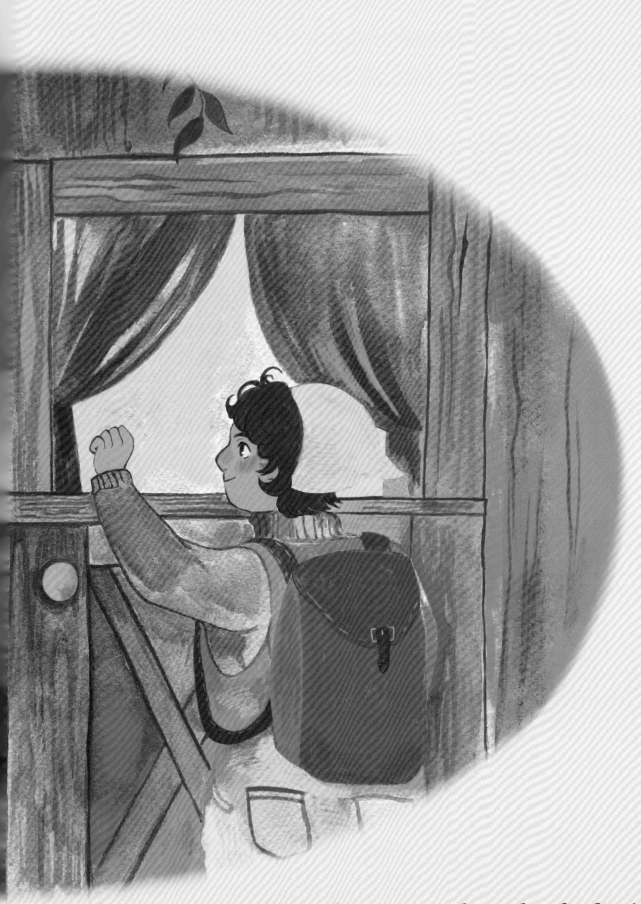

to enter this marvelous herbalist's store.

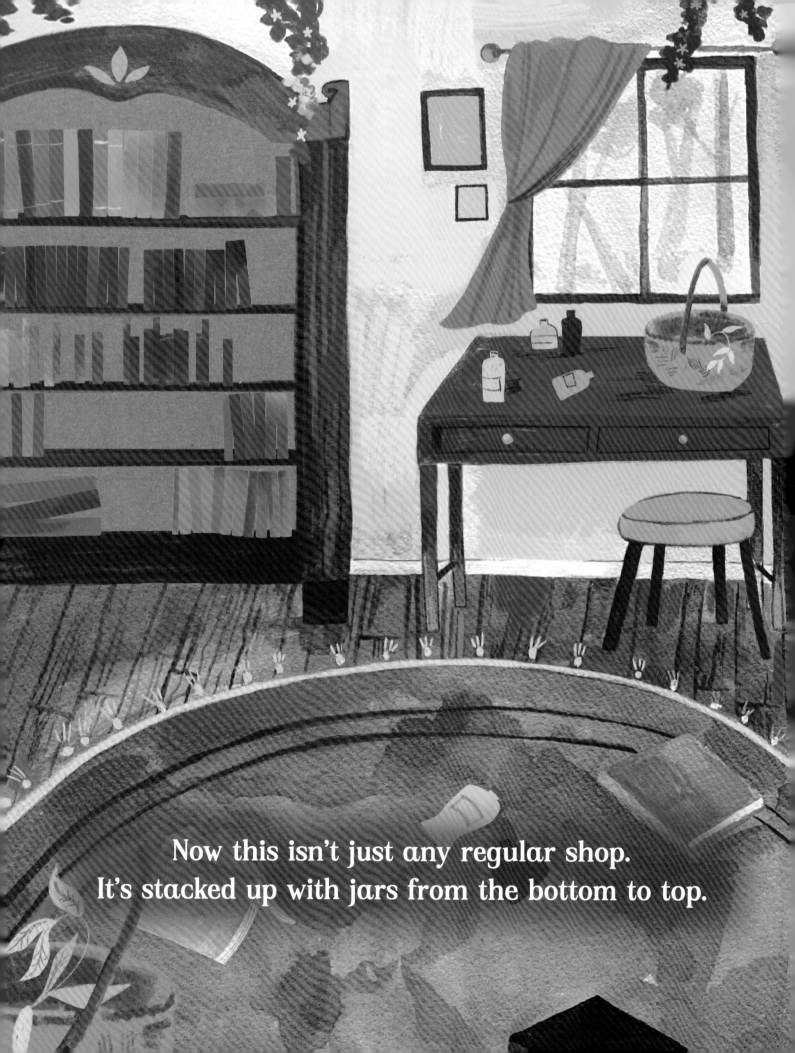

Now this isn't just any regular shop.
It's stacked up with jars from the bottom to top.

Ready to greet you
with knowledge to share,
a faerie stands up
from a small thimble chair.

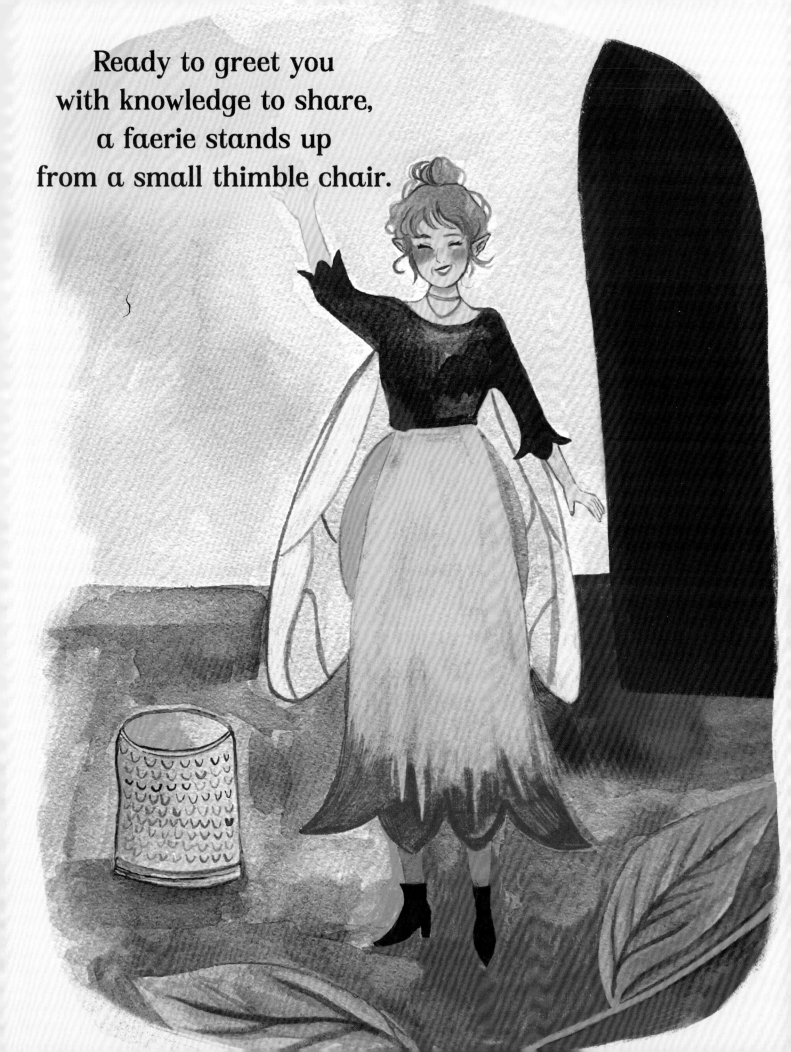

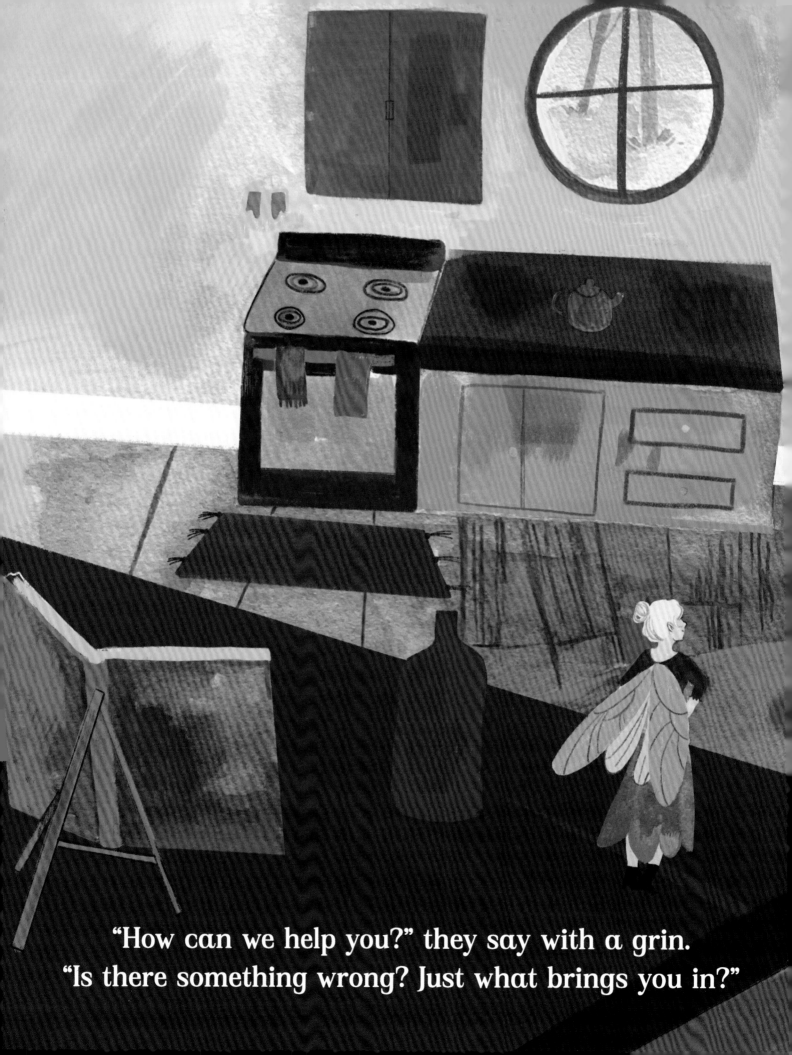

"How can we help you?" they say with a grin.
"Is there something wrong? Just what brings you in?"

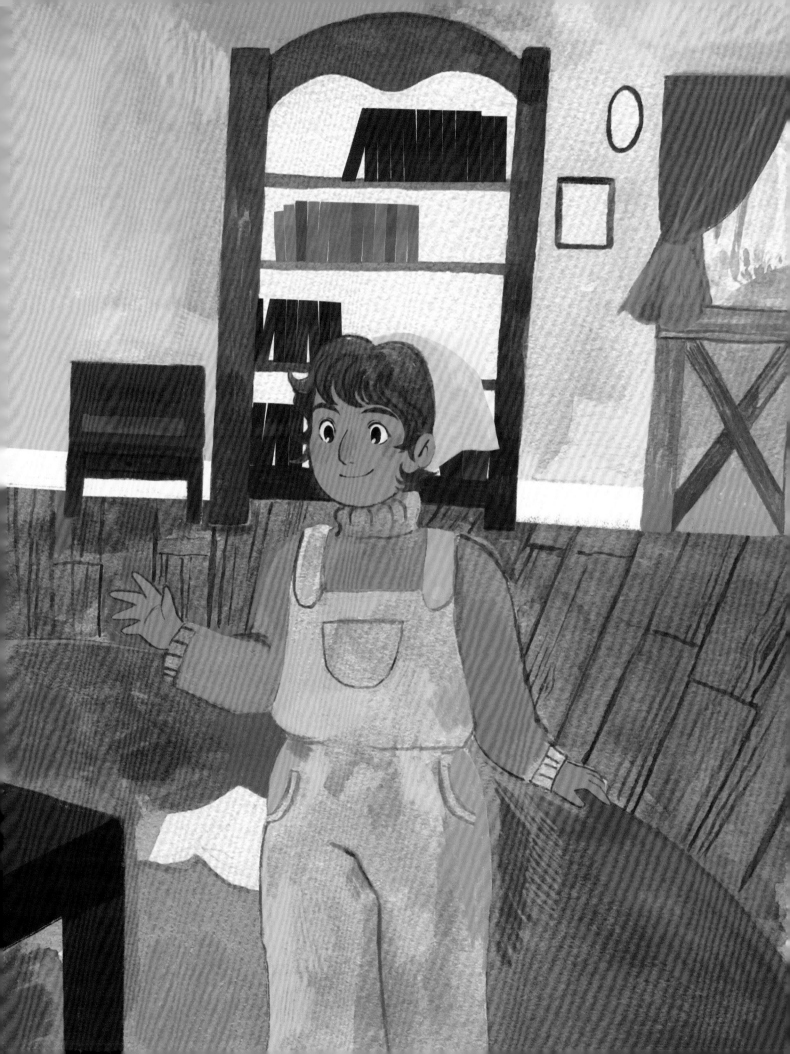

Before you can answer, the bell rings once more
and a line has sprung up from the now-open door.

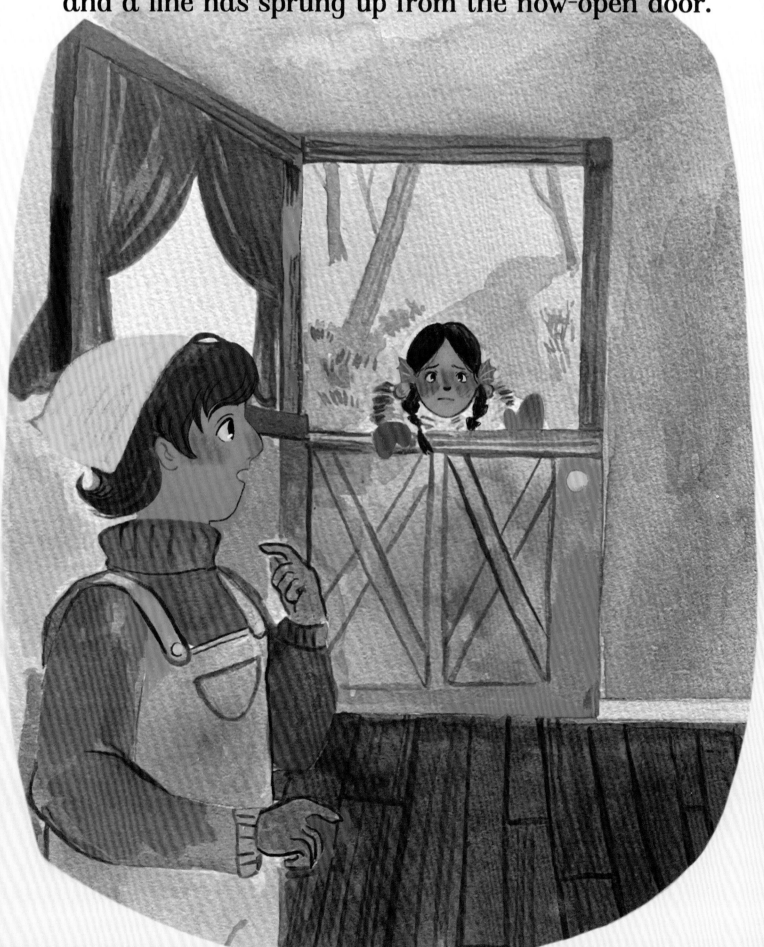

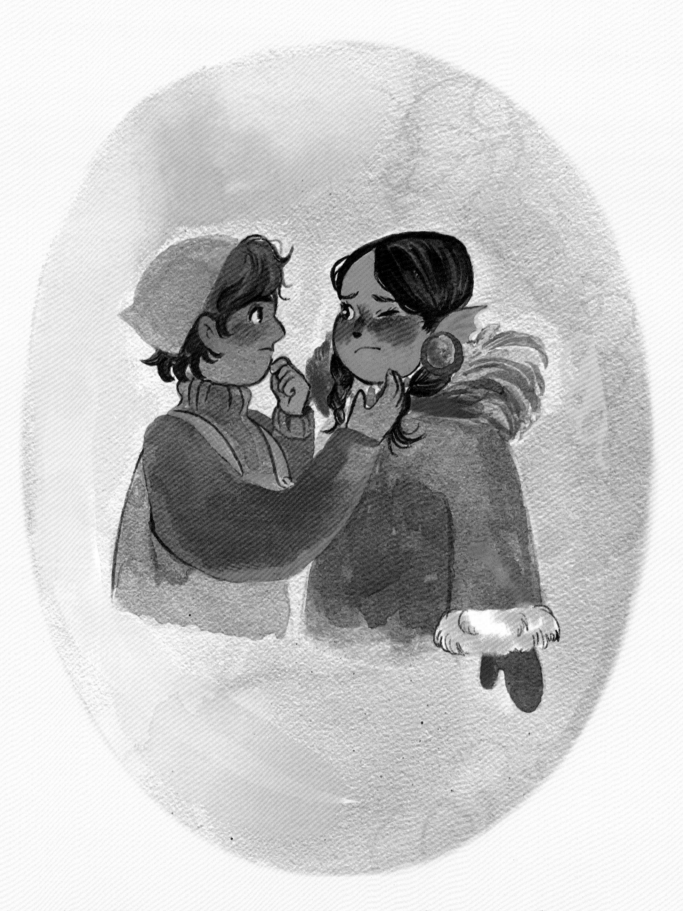

A selkie comes in with a sunburn to show.
She says, "I was trying to get a nice glow!"

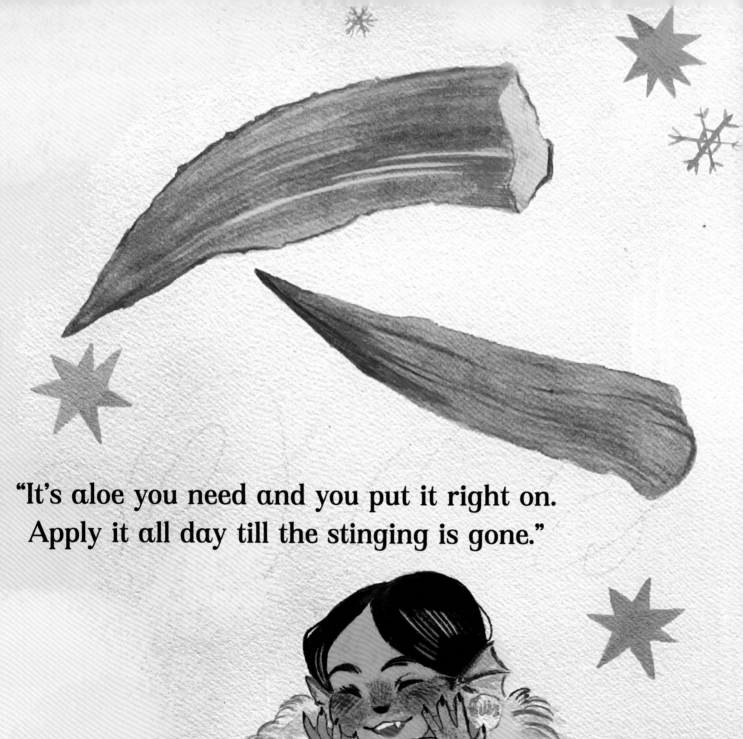

"It's aloe you need and you put it right on.
Apply it all day till the stinging is gone."

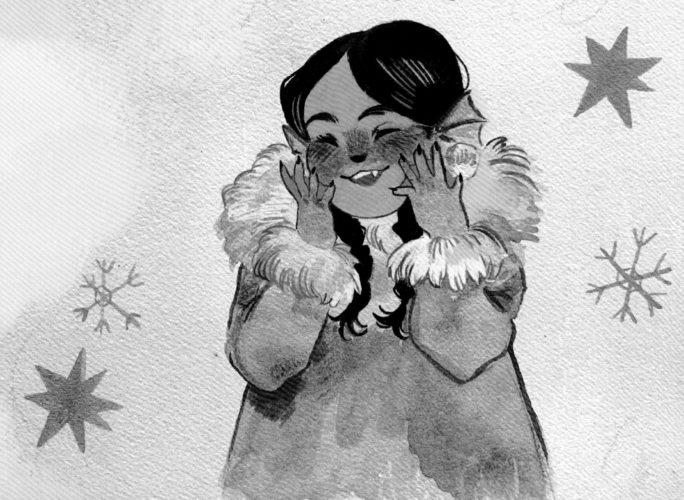

A goblin's up next with a bad stomach ache.
"It's hurting so much, I need something to take!"

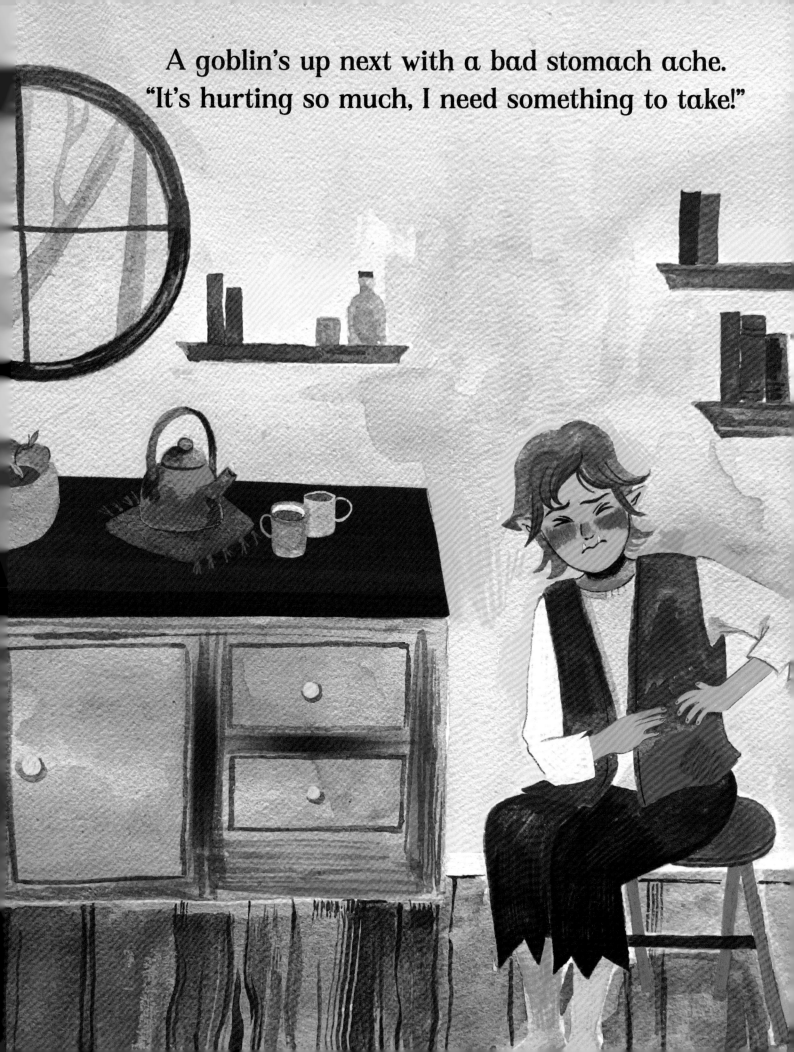

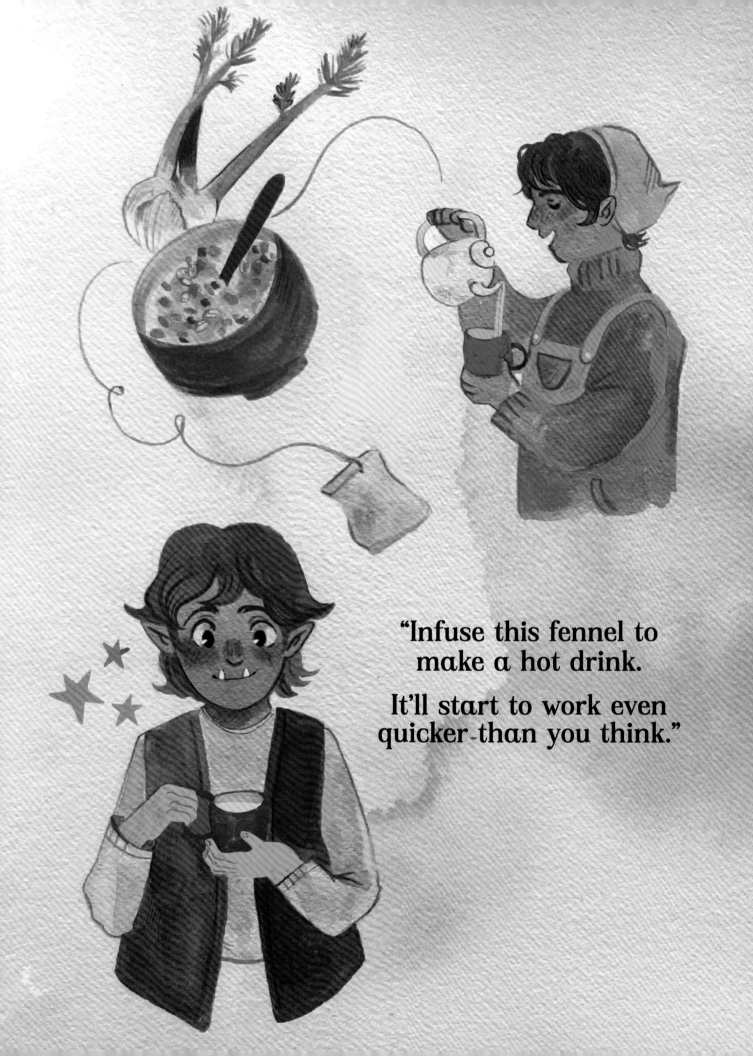

"Infuse this fennel to
make a hot drink.

It'll start to work even
quicker than you think."

A harpy is dealing with terrible stress.
It's causing her headaches. She feels like a mess.

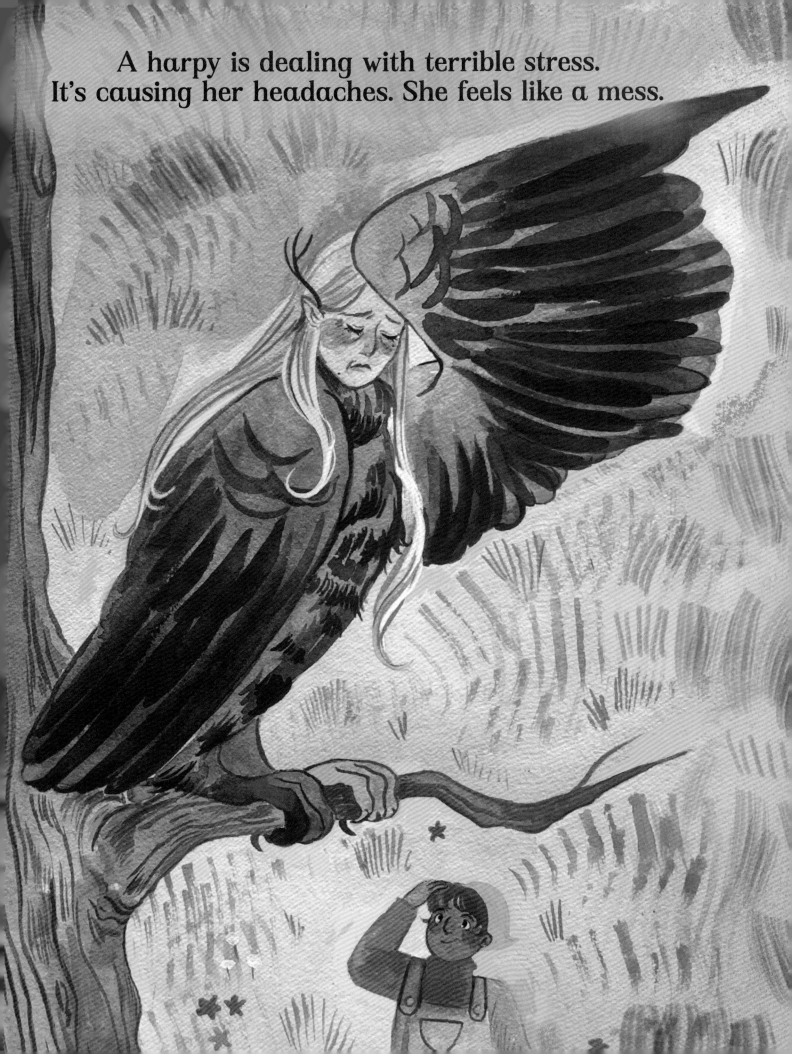

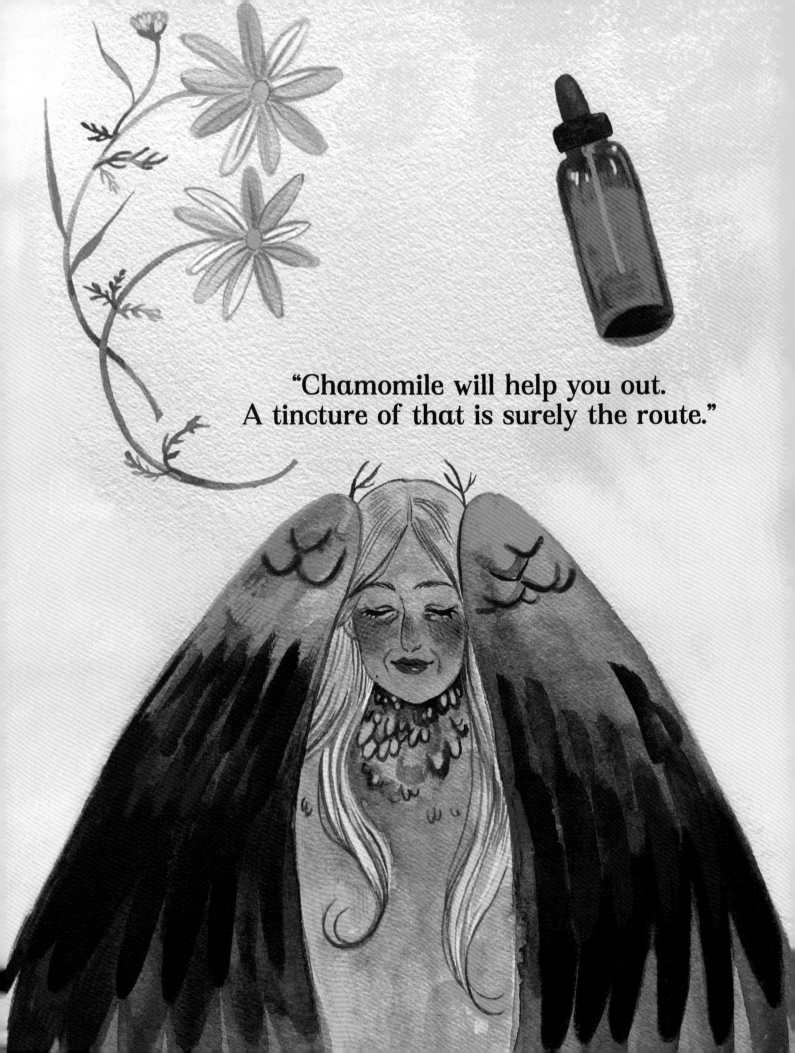

"Chamomile will help you out.
A tincture of that is surely the route."

An elf enters next. She's not looking so bad.
Then she says, "No...I'm just feeling sad."

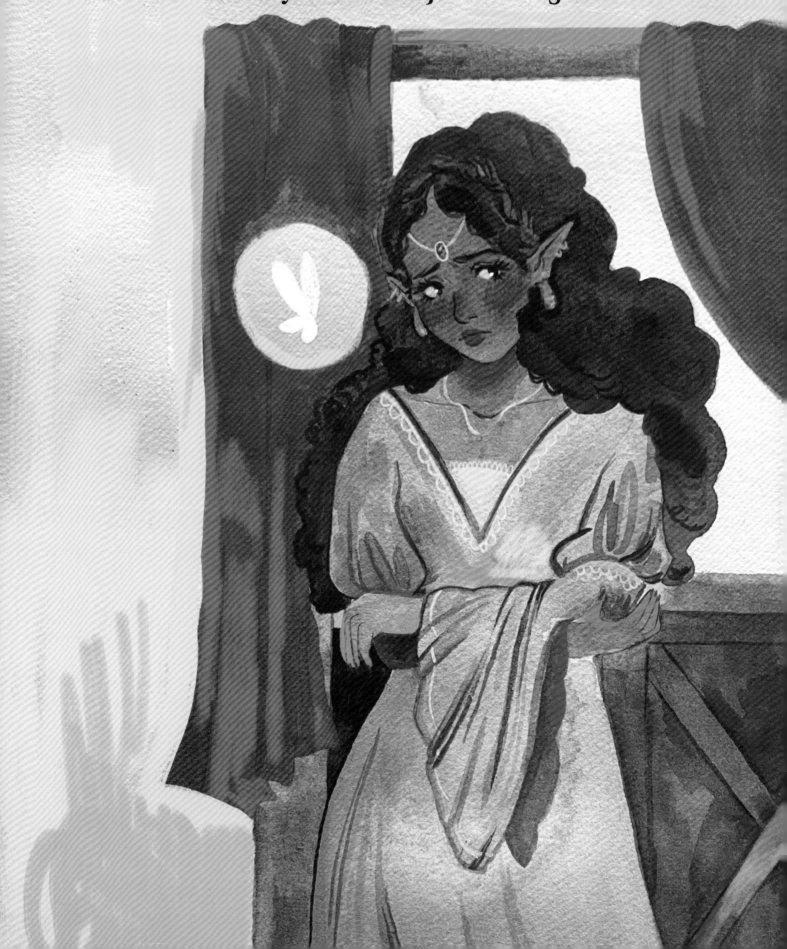

"Hey, sadness is worth treating too.
A tea with St. John's wort for you."

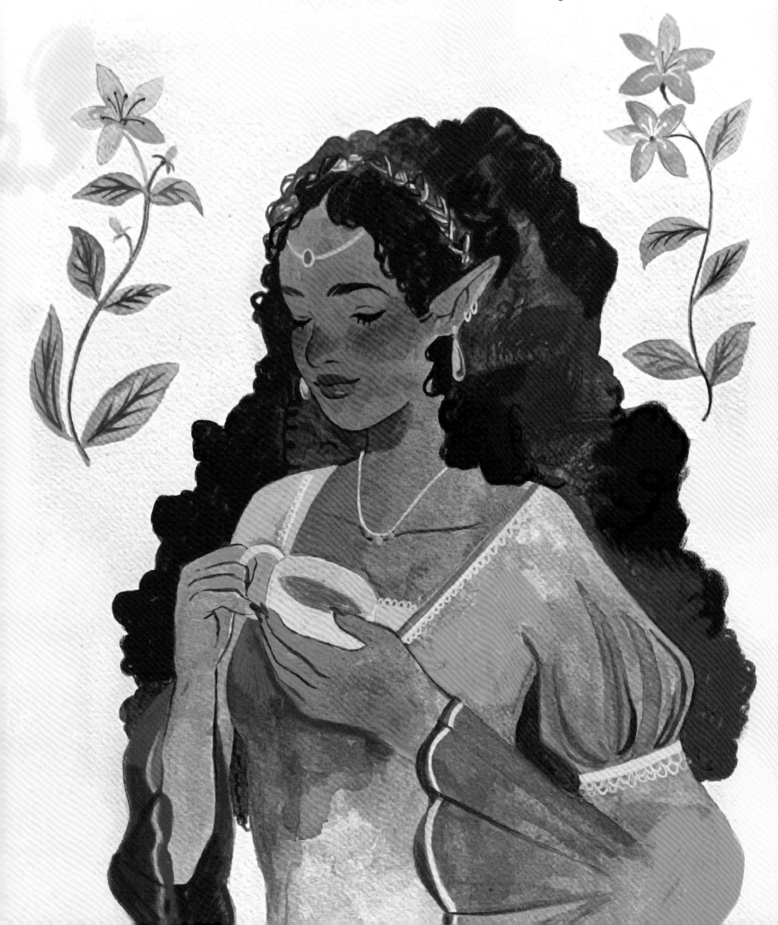

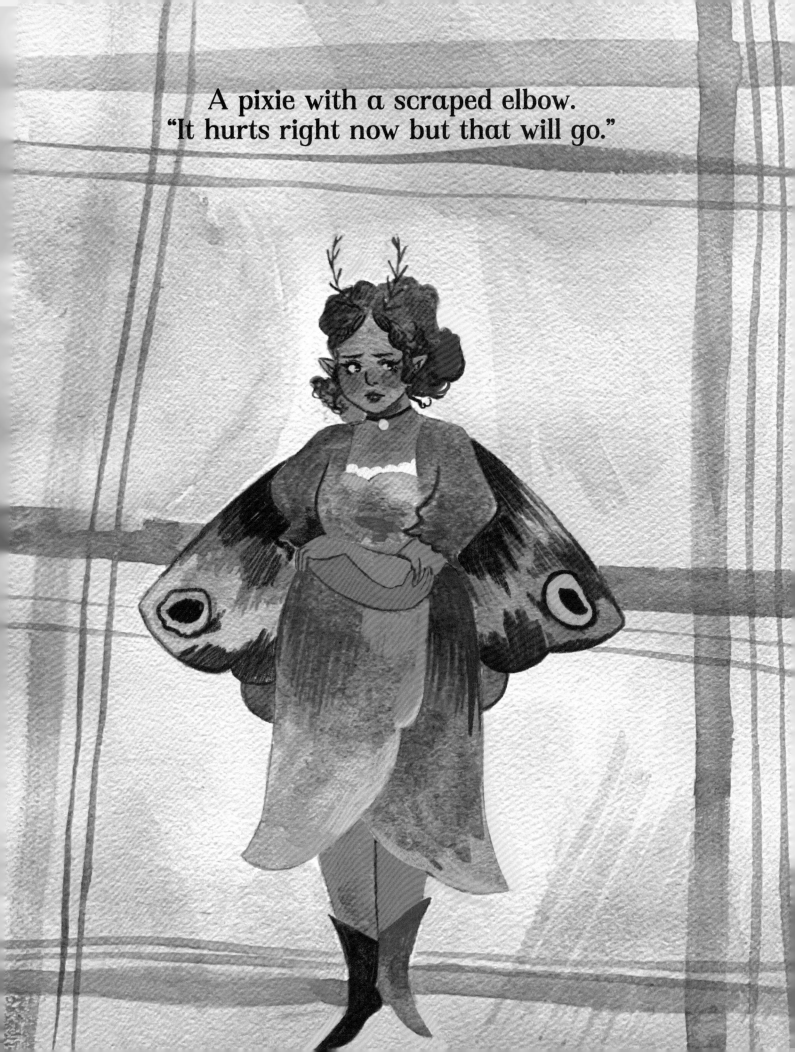

A pixie with a scraped elbow.
"It hurts right now but that will go."

"Pine's the plant to do the trick.
Use this resin. It'll stick!"

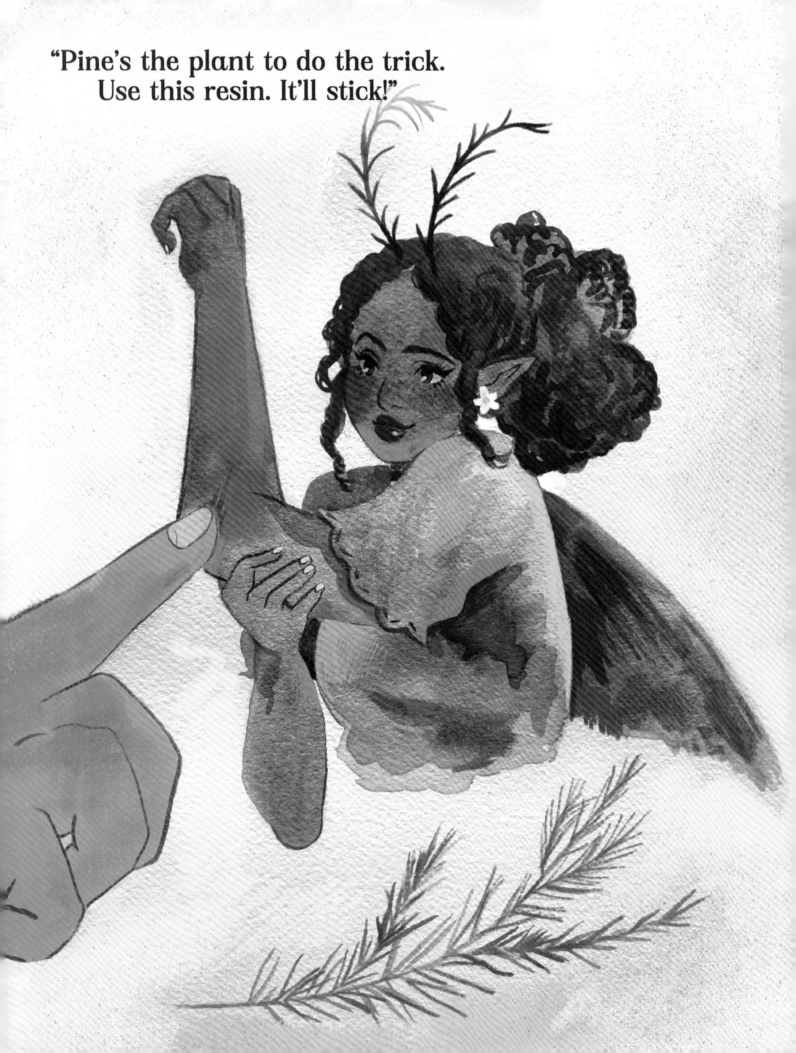

A troll rushes through to the front of the line.
"Sorry for cutting, but I have no time!"

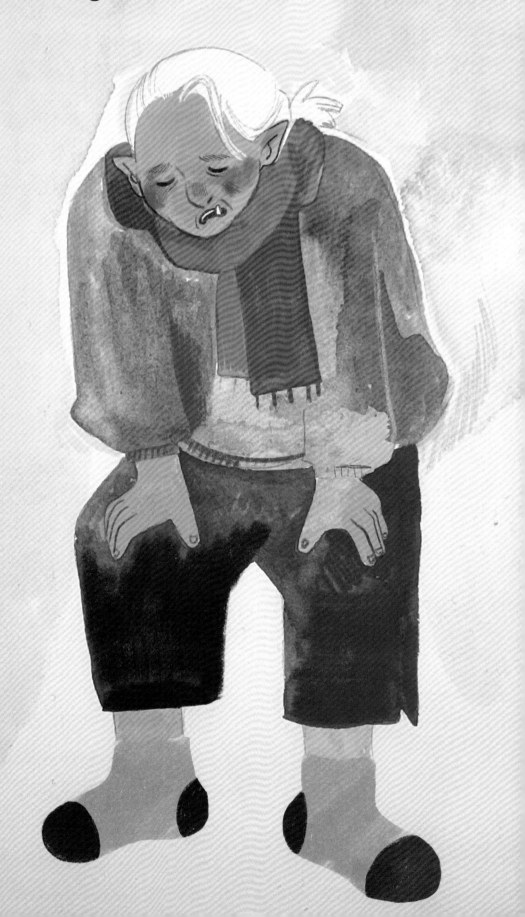

"I have a sore throat
and it doesn't feel nice.
I hurried right in
for I need your advice."

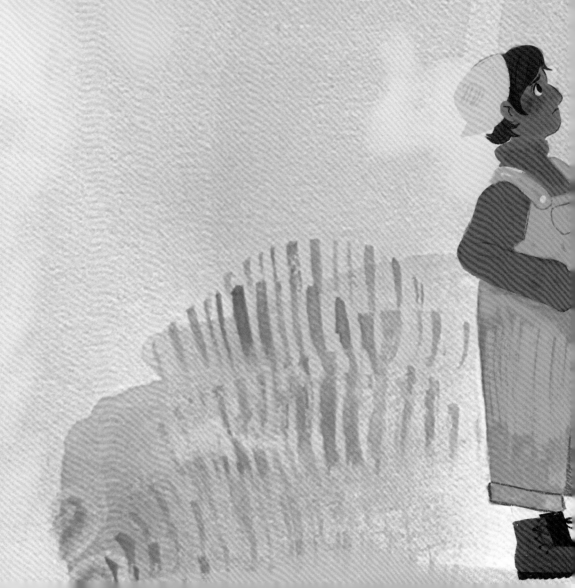

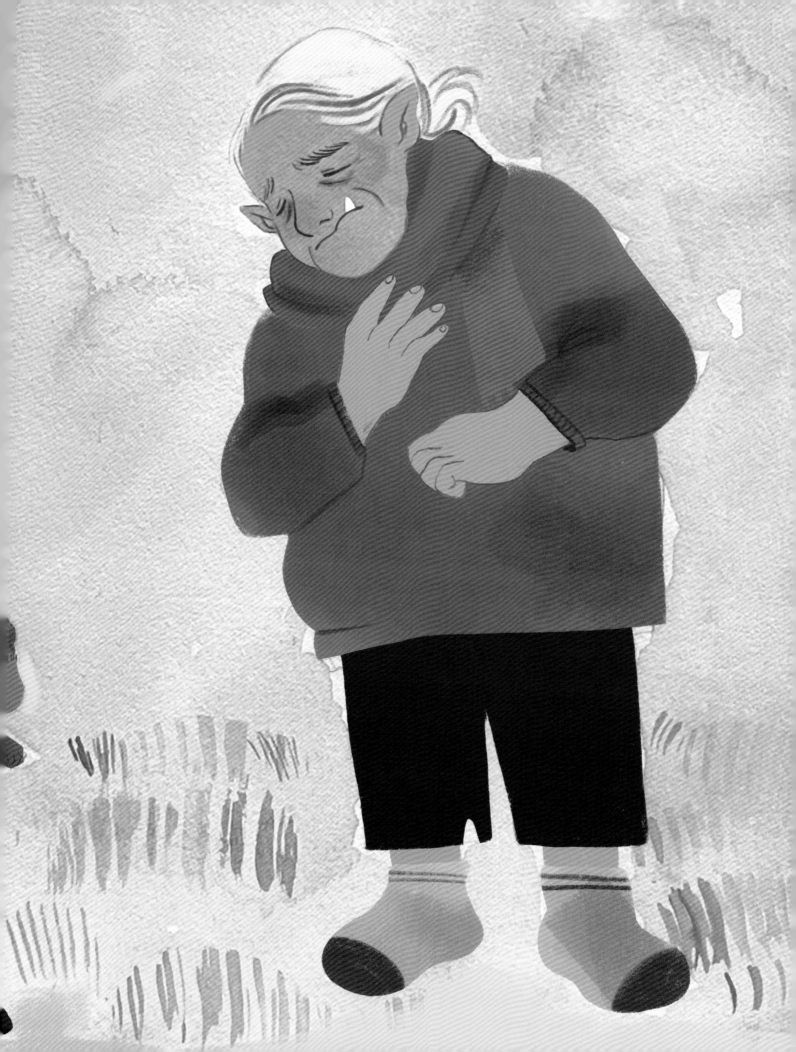

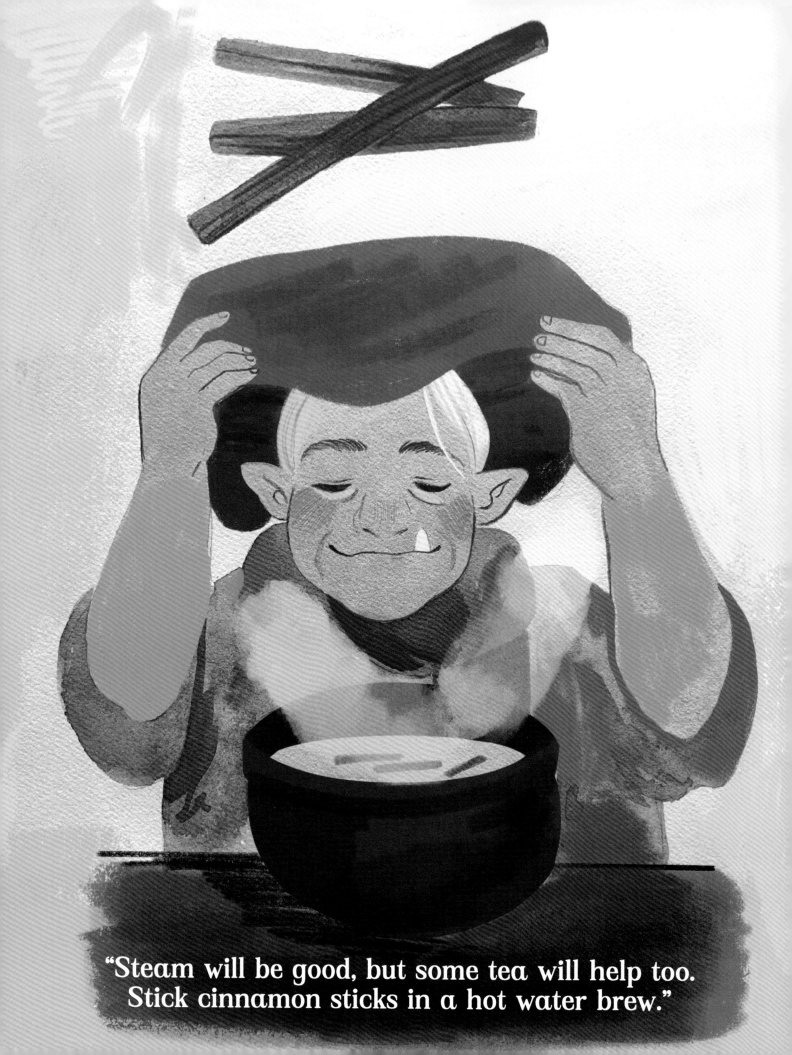

"Steam will be good, but some tea will help too.
Stick cinnamon sticks in a hot water brew."

A kikimora who needs some help to sleep.
"This lavender sachet will make your rest deep."

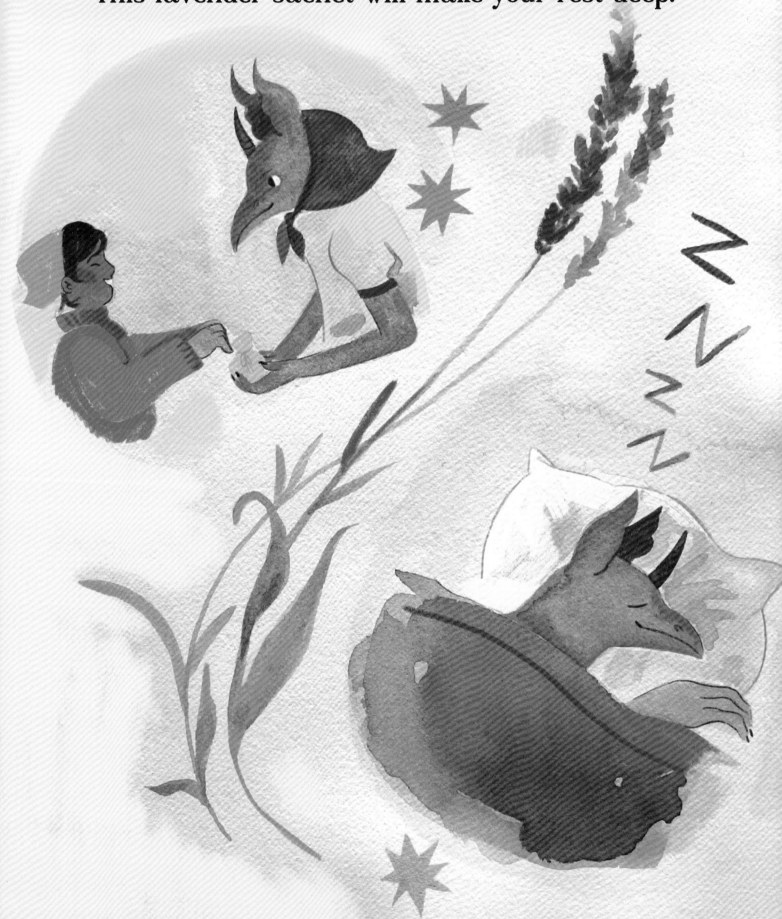

Every ailment fixed right up.
Herbs poured from jars into baskets and cups.

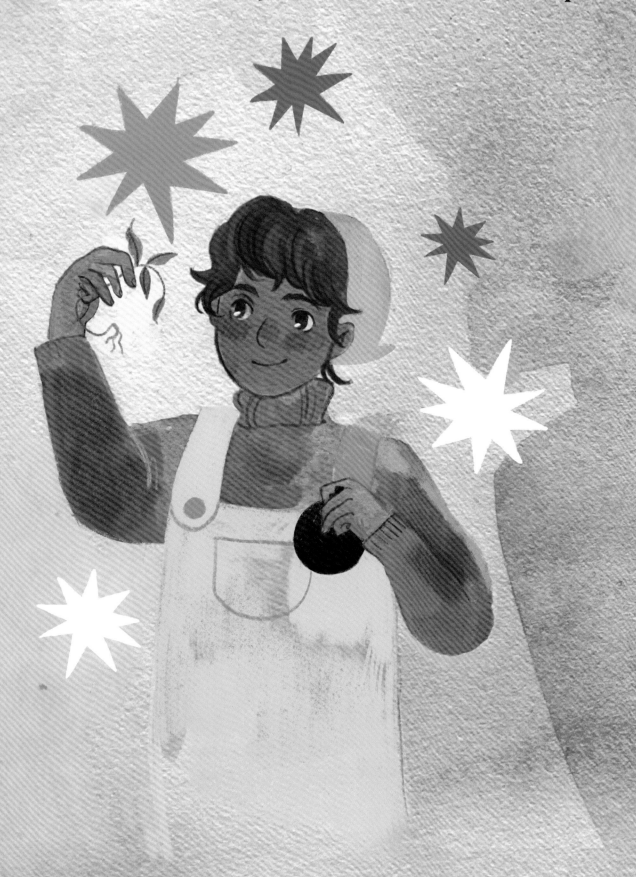

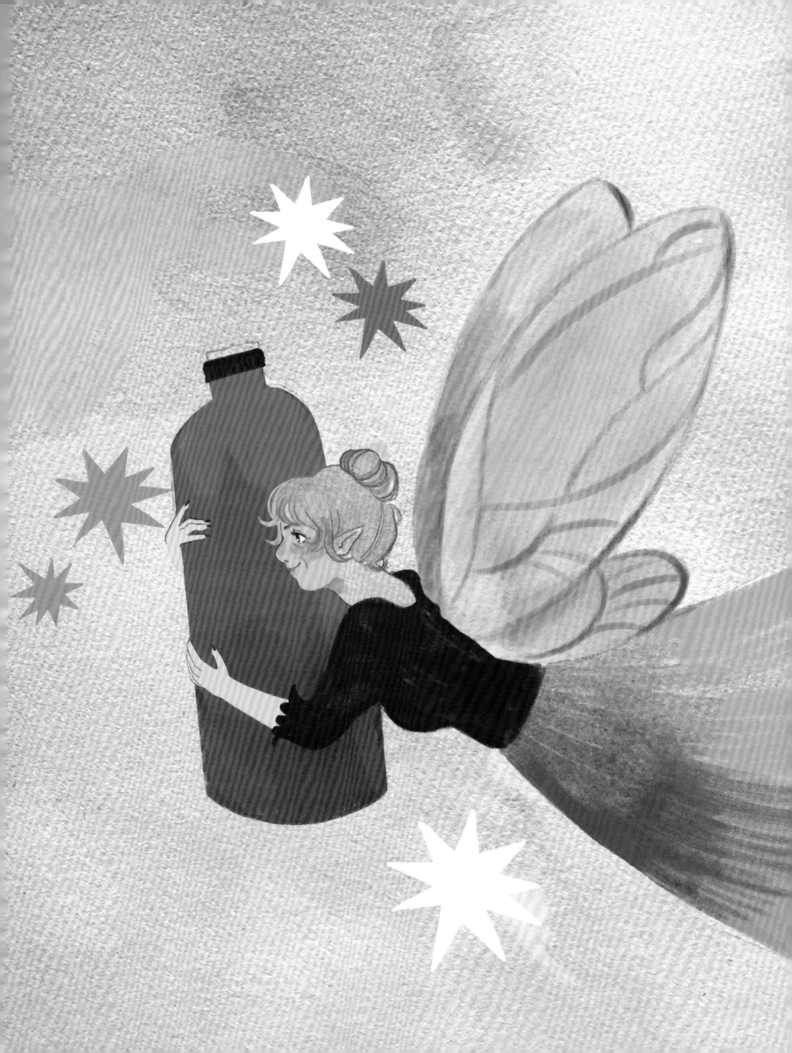

The others have cleared and it's finally your time.
They ask what you need but in fact, "I feel...fine?"

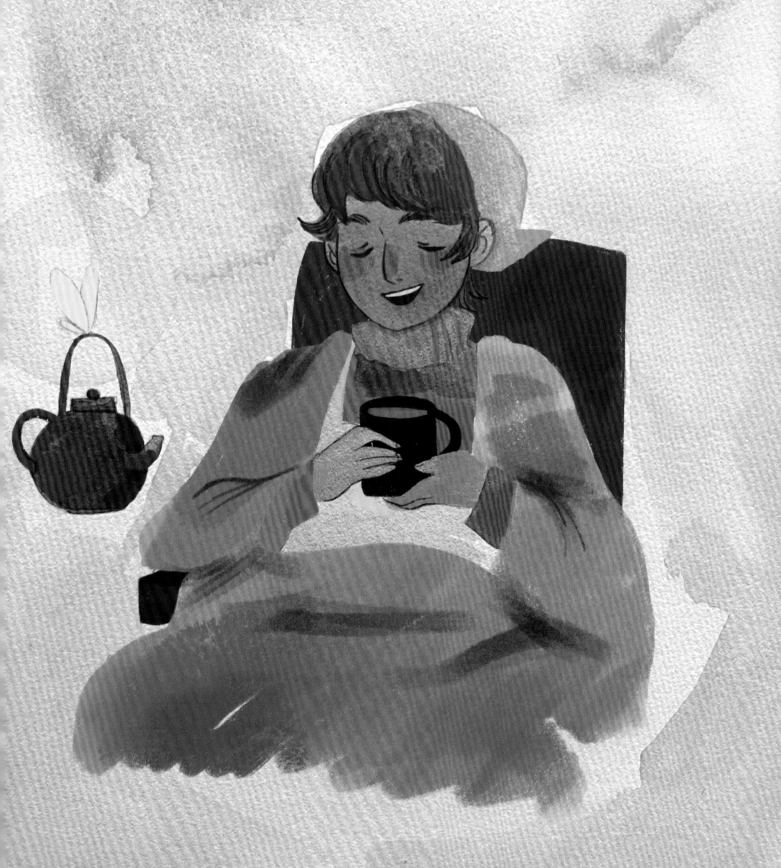

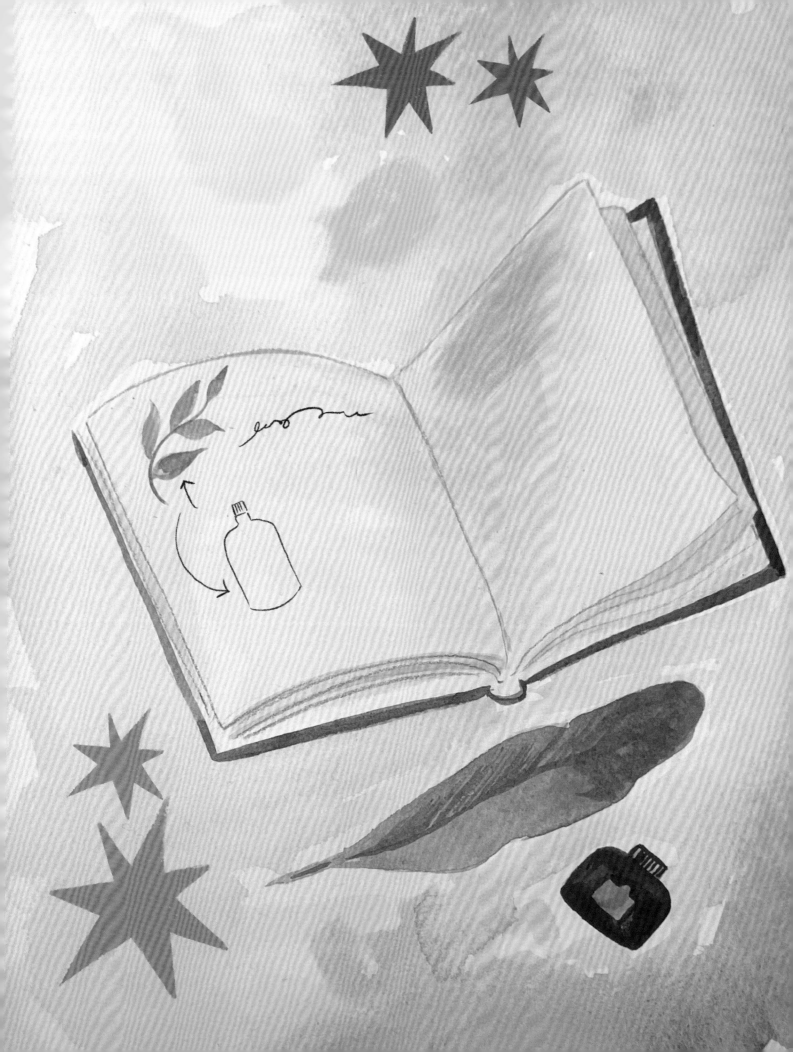

"I was out in the woods and I found this cool door and really, I was just trying to explore.

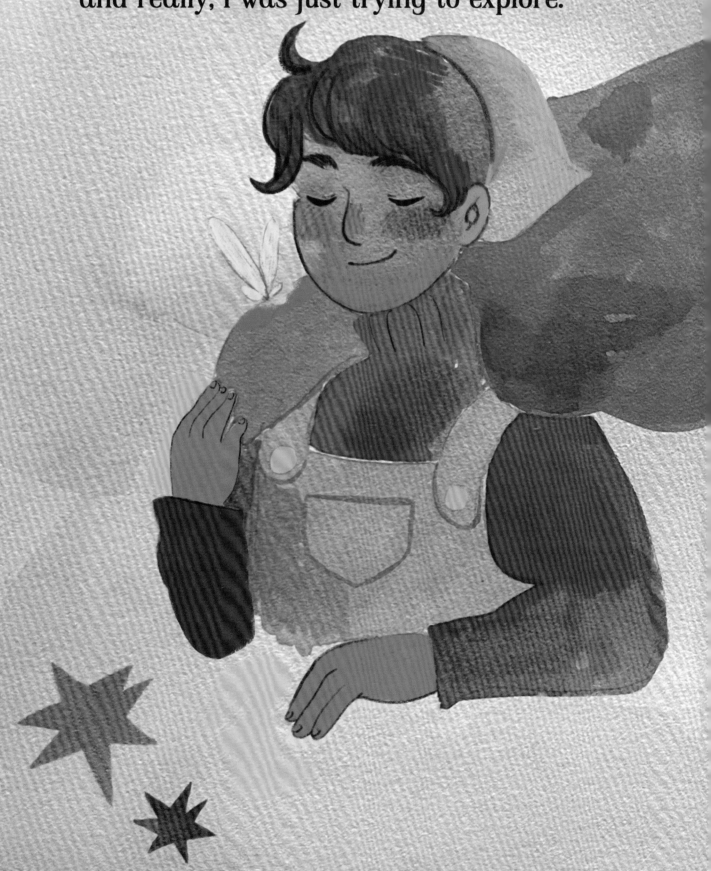

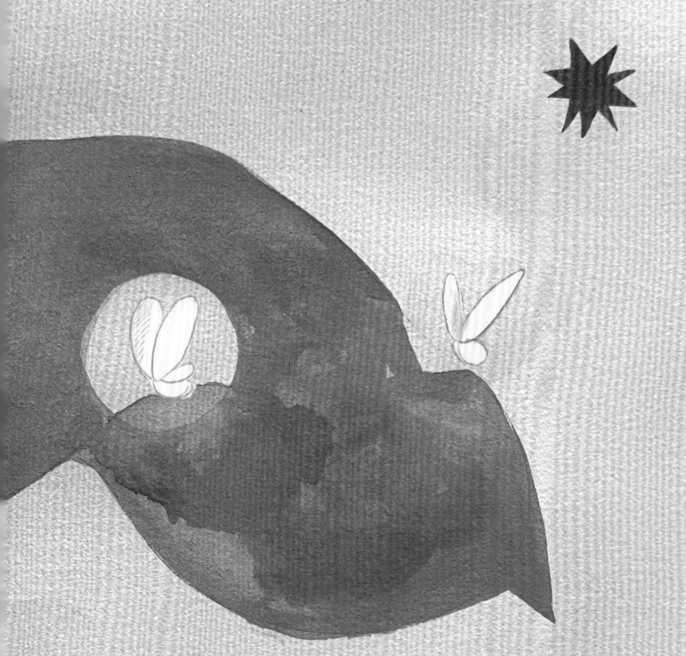

I've learned all about using plants as a cure.
I'll be back, that one's for sure."

But the faeries won't quite let you leave.
They want to give you some reprieve.

"These berries drive sickness away.
Elder keeps your woes at bay."

"Make some syrup, drink a spoon.
Those bad feelings won't catch you soon."

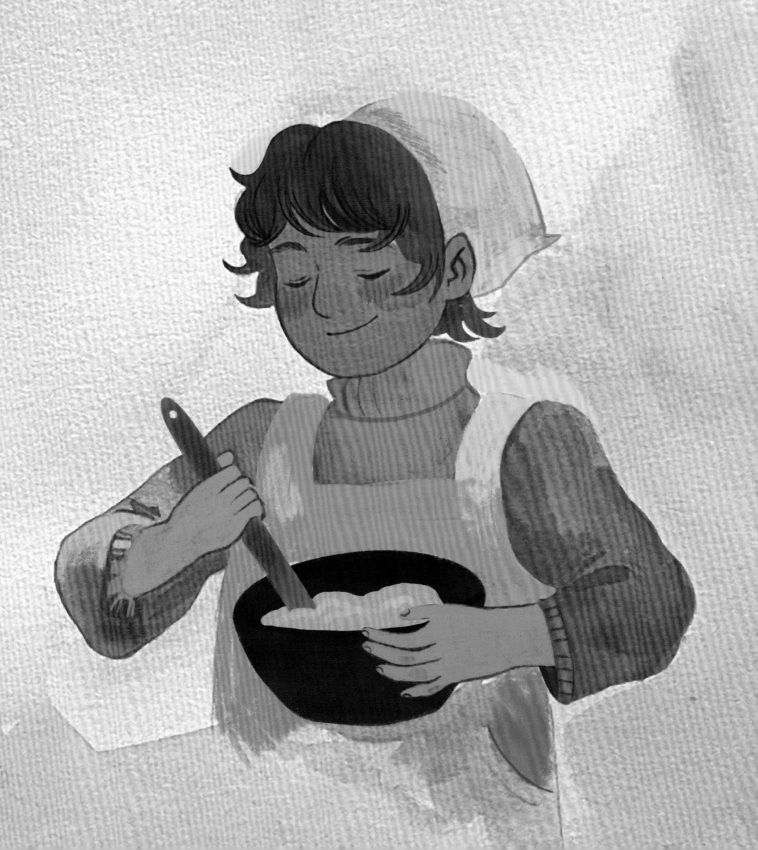

You say goodbye and then you part,
back out into the wooded dark.

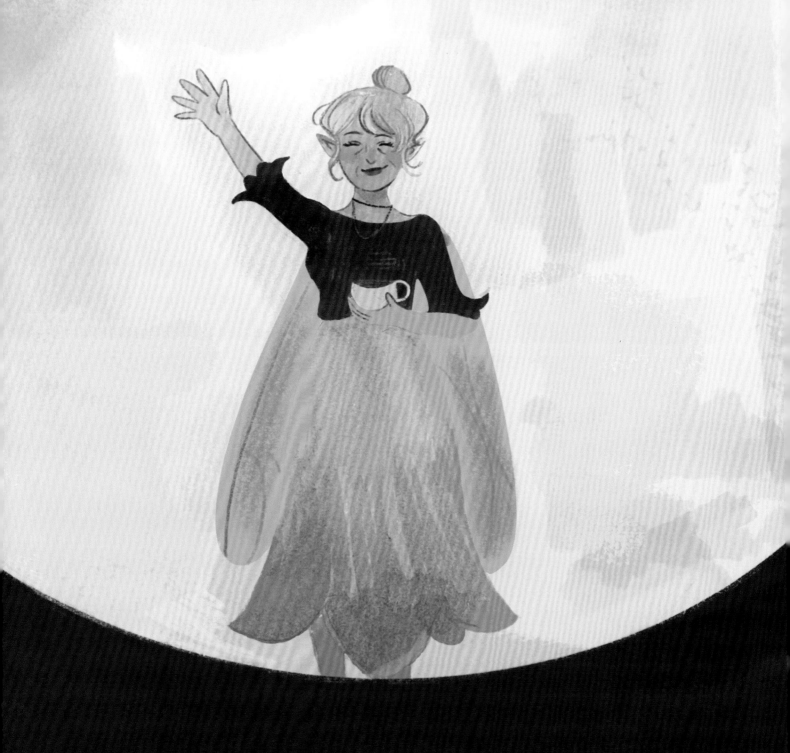

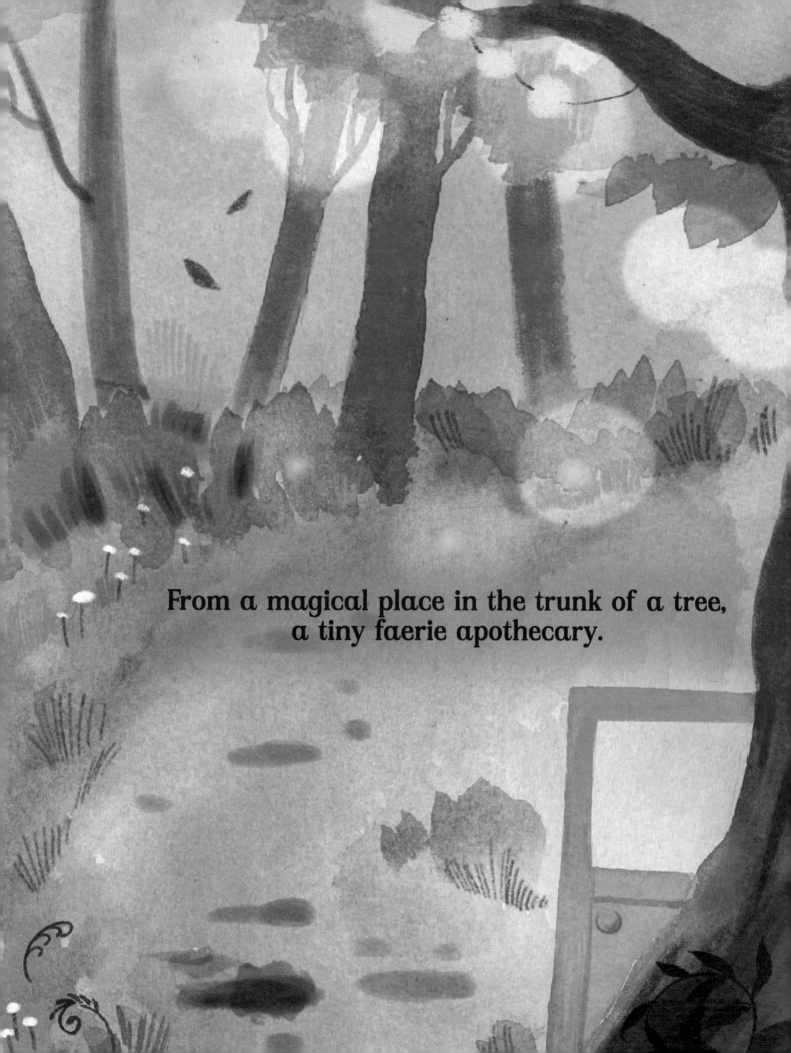

From a magical place in the trunk of a tree,
a tiny faerie apothecary.